yoga

yoga

101 energizing exercises

Susannah Marriott

MQP

Dedication
For Parker, who needs lots of energy to look
after four demanding girls...

Caution
If you are pregnant, have given birth in the last six
weeks, or have a medical condition, such as high
blood pressure, spinal problems, arthritis, or asthma,
consult your medical practitioner or an experienced
remedial yoga teacher before starting yoga practice.
Avoid inverted poses during menstruation.

This book is intended as an informational guide only
and is not to be used as a substitute for professional
medical care or treatment. Neither the author nor the
publisher can be held responsible for any damage,
injury, or otherwise resulting from the use of the
information in this book.

Published by MQ Publications Limited
12 The Ivories, 6-8 Northampton Street
London N1 2HY
Tel: 020 7359 2244
Fax: 020 7359 1616
email: mail@mqpublications.com
website: www.mqpublications.com

Series Editor: Karen Ball, MQ Publications
Editorial Director: Ljiljana Baird, MQ Publications
Senior Designer: Victoria Bevan, MQ Publications
Photography by Mike Prior
Design by Balley Design Associates

ISBN 1-84072-536-2

Printed in France by *Partenaires-Livres*® (JL)

1 3 5 7 9 0 8 6 4 2

contents

Introduction

We all crave the sensations energy brings: feeling alert, able to cope with any problem, poised, strong, and on top of the world. When energy flows, everything flows: creative powers, charisma, humor, and coping mechanisms; the body seems to move with effortless grace, attuned with the mind and in harmony with the environment. Yoga can bring you this. My favorite yoga classes are evening sessions after a heavy day attempting to work while caring for a baby and two young children. I can hardly drag myself to class after the maelstrom of breastfeeding and bedtime. All I want to do is doze in front of the TV with a glass of wine. But when I emerge from the energetic, physically taxing class two hours later, I feel tall, capable, and full of energy, fired up for anything and yet filled with a spacious sense of calm.

When yoga teachers talk about energy, they refer not only to that instant physical buzz that results from food, exercise, or a good night's rest, but to a more considered subtle form, known as prana. Prana, meaning life-force and breath, is part of everything in the universe: it animates not only human beings and animals, but the wind, rocks, trees, and foodstuff. When we breathe or absorb food, we take within us this energy of the universe in an intense cosmic union. The energy travels along some 72,000 invisible pathways, or nadis, in the subtle body to keep all the body's systems functioning at their best. The most important nadi, the sushumna, runs alongside the spine, from pelvis to crown. Seven energy centers, or chakras, sit along the sushumna, where nadis meet, trapping and directing energy to circulate throughout the body. By practicing yoga postures, asana, and breathing techniques, pranayama, we clear blockages in this flow of vital energy, and ensure that each part of the body, joints to glands, organs to muscles, bones to ligaments, exists in a state of balance. When life-force flows in this way, we feel as we should—full of life, wellbeing, and vitality—and good health ensues. Certain asanas and breathing techniques, carried out under the guidance of a spiritual master, are said to rouse the dormant very powerful divine energy force within each of us known as kundalini.

Use the ideas in this book to rediscover your innate energy and get it flowing. When you're stressed out and have lost it; when you're so tired you can hardly speak; when your mind loses its focus and your whole body aches, remember that yoga can lift you. Let the postures relax your tension and realign your body so energy flows anew; let the breathwork shut down your ties to the world, giving your mental powers time to regroup. Tune out of stress and fatigue with yoga and you will find yourself realigning in mindful meditation with the energy of the universe.

Tips for good practice

- Wear loose clothing—track pants and a vest or T-shirt.
- For breathwork and meditation, slip on socks and a shawl or sweatshirt to keep the body warm.
- Work with bare feet and invest in a sticky yoga mat.
- After a heavy meal, wait two hours before practicing yoga.
- Warm up briefly before beginning a pose: circle your shoulders, neck, hips, knees, and ankles; shake out the arms and legs, and stretch the large muscles in these limbs.
- Instead of trying consciously to achieve something, just focus on the pose.
- Expect to feel stiffness after yoga if you do not practice regularly. Start gently, and keep up the practice—with regular sessions 2–3 times a week, stiffness will disappear after 2 or 3 weeks.

Rewiring the brain

Whether your sagging energy levels result
from lack of sleep, overwork, or sheer stress,
yoga can provide a solution.

1 After a sleepless night

❶ Lie on your back, legs apart, feet dropping out. Relax your arms away from your sides, palms up. Lift your head, align with your body, and replace on the mat. Close your eyes.

❷ Tense and relax every part of the body. Work upward, tightening and releasing your feet, calves, thighs and buttocks, abdomen and chest, hands and arms, shoulders and neck.

❸ Screw up your face, then yawn widely. Release, relaxing the jaw, forehead, and mouth, your tongue, ears, and back of head.

❹ Focus on deepening your breath, then relax the mind, watching thoughts pass with disinterest. Remain in the pose for 5–10 minutes. Stretch before sitting up.

2 To refresh the brain

❶ Stand tall in Tadasana (see page 30). Inhaling, take your arms overhead, shoulders relaxing away from the ears. Hold for a couple of breath cycles. Exhaling, pivot from the hips to stretch forward, as if trying to touch a far-off wall with the tips of your fingers.

❷ Bend your knees and place your torso on your thighs: stomach on upper thighs, chest on lower thighs. Place your hands by your feet. Work for 30 seconds on straightening your legs with each out-breath, ensuring no gap develops between chest and legs. With each in-breath, take refreshing oxygen to tight areas. Come up, head last, on an inhalation.

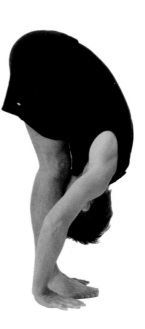

3 For mental invigoration

❶ Standing in Tadasana (see page 30), jump your feet 3–4ft apart. Inhaling, raise your arms overhead, stretching from ankles to fingertips.

❷ Exhaling, extend forward, pivoting from the hips and maintaining the stretch along the entire spine. Place your palms flat on the floor and hang between your legs, anchoring on all parts of the feet.

❸ Hold for 30 seconds or more, crown of the head resting on the floor, if possible, lengthening the spine and back of the legs. Let each exhalation pull the abdomen in and up. Inhale to come up.

4 To focus attention

❶ Standing in Tadasana (page 30), feet hip-width apart, take your weight on to the right foot. Lift your left foot and press the sole into the inner ankle, calf, or thigh of the standing leg, knee outward. Bring palms together in prayer position in front of your chest.

❷ Root your standing foot down, then lift through the ankle, calf, and thigh. Lengthen through your torso as if your pelvis is weighted. Open your chest, squaring shoulders with hips. With chin tucked toward the throat, pull up through the back of the skull, as if suspended by a string.

❸ When stable, inhale and extend your arms overhead, fingers pressing together, shoulders releasing from ears. Hold for 30 seconds or more. Repeat on the other leg.

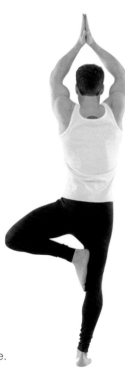

5 To ground intellectual energy

❶ Standing in Tadasana (page 30) with feet hip-width apart, imagine growing roots into the ground. Feel yourself anchored to the earth.

❷ Sway from side to side, then increase the movements, making large circles in both directions with feet glued to the spot. Feel nervous tension earthing into the ground.

❸ Come back to center, adopt Vrkasana (page 13), taking the lifted leg into half-lotus position, placing the foot in the groin crease of the standing leg, knee pressing down.

❹ Hold for 30 seconds or more, feeling the strength of the standing leg. If desired, take your arms overhead, inhaling. Visualize them as branches growing out into the air element as your trunk stays rooted in the earth. Breathe deeply.

6 Memory sharpener

❶ Standing in Tadasana (page 30), extend back your right toes and straighten the leg. Lift the leg as if your back thigh is heavy, pointing your toes at the wall behind you, hips level.

❷ Rotate your left arm so the palm faces backward and, exhaling, lift the arm overhead, fingers pointing up, shoulder dropping away from the ear.

❸ Raise your right arm to the side without lifting your shoulder, outstretched fingers at a 45° angle to the wall. Hold for up to 30 seconds, maintaining focus on all three planes simultaneously. Repeat to the other side.

7 Cross-patterning the brain

❶ Start on hands and knees, shoulders over wrists, knees under hips, looking down so the spine is aligned from its base to the crown of the head.

❷ Inhaling, lift your left arm and right leg. Exhaling, stretch your fingertips forward and point your toes away. Hold for a few breath cycles, fingers and toes level, feeling the stretch diagonally through the spine.

❸ Exhaling, bring the limbs back down to the hands and knees position. Repeat with opposite limbs. Repeat the exercise 5 times.

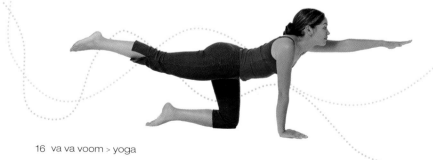

8 Hangover blitz

❶ Sit tall in Dandasana (page 32), toes and knees pointing up, palms pressing down. Bend your right leg, knee dropping outward, and bring the sole to rest against the opposite thigh.

❷ Inhaling, raise your arms overhead, shoulders dropping. Exhaling, hinge forward from level hips and, looking forward, catch your outstretched calf, ankle, or toes.

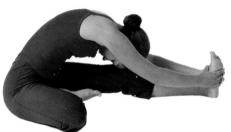

❸ With each exhalation, bring your spine forward and down, so that eventually you place your abdomen, chest, and finally your forehead on the outstretched leg. Hold for 30 seconds or more, sinking into the stretch with each out-breath and taking fresh oxygen to tight areas with each inhalation. Inhale to come up. Repeat on the other leg.

9 For the morning after

❶ Lie on your front, legs outstretched and touching, arms by your sides (palms up), forehead on the floor.

❷ Rotate your arms so your chest and shoulders are square to the floor, and your palms face down. On an exhalation, stretch your right leg away from you, pointing your toes at the wall behind.

❸ Feeling your thigh heavy and keeping your leg straight, inhale, raising your calf as if trying to place your sole on the ceiling. Isolate the stretch in the buttock, keeping the spine relaxing downward. Hold for a few breath cycles, lowering on an exhalation. Repeat on the other leg.

10 Boosting brainpower

❶ Sit with buttocks and back against a wall, legs outstretched. Swivel to one side, buttocks still in contact with the wall, then turn on to your back, both buttocks touching the wall, spine flat to the mat.

❷ Work to straighten the legs against the wall with each out-breath, pressing through the heels and both sides of the soles, as if supporting a heavy weight.

❸ If desired, inhale and stretch your arms above your chest. Hold, relaxing the shoulders and small of the back into the mat, then slowly lower your arms to rest beyond your head. With each out-breath work to keep the entire spine on the mat. With each in-breath feel your back and shoulders spread outward. Hold for 3 minutes or more.

11 For clearer vision

❶ Lie on your back, legs outstretched, arms by your side, palms down. Slide each palm beneath your pelvis, buttocks resting on the back of the hands.

❷ Inhaling, press on your elbows to lift your torso. Extend through your upper arms and shoulders to open your chest to the ceiling. Take your head back and rest it on the crown. Look backward, eyes open wide, and point your toes toward your knees.

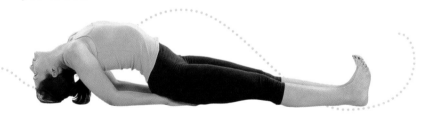

❸ Hold for 30 seconds or more; with each exhalation feel the chest broaden and energy generating in the throat, heart, and crown of the head. Relax down on an exhalation.

12 For concentration

❶ Sit comfortably upright with legs crossed. Stretch your palms and fingers out, then rest your hands, palms upward, loosely on your knees. Bring the tips of the first finger and thumb on each hand to touch lightly. Stretch out your three remaining digits, fingers touching.

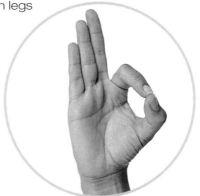

❷ Close your eyes and focus on your breath, seeing it deepen and slow as you watch it moving in and out, and feeling calmness and concentration fill you. Work for 3 minutes or more.

13 Springcleaning the brain

❶ Sitting on your heels, if possible, palms on your knees or thighs, take a long, full breath in through your nostrils. Let it drop into the lower part of the abdomen, as if filling a balloon from the bottom up.

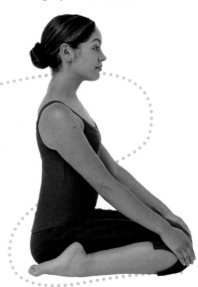

❷ With mouth closed, expel the inhalation by pulling your navel toward your spine sharply three or more times. Feel stale air leaving the body, cleansing on its way the back of the throat and top of the palate. Relax your abdomen to let the in-breath come naturally and smoothly. Repeat 3 rounds of 10 breaths, returning to regular breathing between each round.

14 To quiet the brain

❶ Sit in a comfortable upright position, hands on your thighs or knees, palms upward. Close your eyes and start to notice your breathing.

❷ Reside within, simply watching your breathing become deeper and longer, losing all thoughts. Thoughts will occur, but don't follow them: imagine your mind as a blue sky, and the thoughts as clouds passing. Ignore sounds, too, drawing within, away from all your senses.

❸ Work for 3–5 minutes. After finishing, sit silently, becoming attuned to the outside world, but retaining an inner awareness of composure, lack of worries, and peace.

15 Thoughtful energy

In each yoga asana, let your entire body and mind inhabit the pose in order to absorb its unique expression of energy. Feel every inch of yourself becoming part of the posture; not just those bits of the body that are moving. Sense the opposite side of the body, think about what's happening to your internal organs, be aware of the way your skin folds and stretches from the crown of your head to your little toes. And engage your senses, too. Feel how the pose affects your eyes, ears, nose, and mouth—get to know what each asana feels like in order to find its energy.

Reviving the body

Sense the rejuvenating effect of even the smallest movement carried out with awareness. For when you take your attention to parts of the body that are moving, your breath follows, and with it prana, the stuff of life.

16 Lively up yourself

❶ Lie on your back in Savasana (page 10). Take time to release tension from every part of your body, and with it, any mental tension you may have.

❷ Keeping your eyes closed, start to roll on to one side, making the movement so slow that it is hardly noticeable. Work as if you have all day to reach your side. Imagine each cell within initiating the movement and providing the propulsion.

❸ Once you reach one side, complete the movement by rolling on to your front, again working so slowly that you remain unsure whether you are moving or not. Treat the end of one action as the start of the next to keep your energy free-flowing.

17 Couch potato antidote

❶ Lie on your back, knees bent and feet flat on the floor, arms by your side, slightly away from the body. Stretch on to tiptoes, then place your heels down, anchoring through the big and little toes and the width of the heels.

❷ Inhaling, focus on your pelvis. Feel it soften and, exhaling, give the bones to the floor. Release any gripping, letting the small of your back drop.

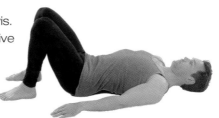

❸ Now focus on your shoulder blades. Exhaling, feel them melt into the floor, giving up ingrained patterns of holding.

❹ On another out-breath, slide your shoulders away from your ears so that the back of your arms rest comfortably on the floor. Feel your head heavy, back of the neck dropping. Rest here for 3 minutes or more, watching your breath.

18 Foot revival

❶ Stand in Tadasana (page 30). Inhaling, raise your arms overhead, rise up on tiptoes, and hold, gathering tension in your calves.

❷ Then, exhaling all tension, fall down on to flat feet, making a bang on the floor and letting your arms flop downward. Repeat 3 or 5 times.

19 Absorbing earth energy

❶ Stand with feet hip-width apart, parallel on the outer edge (pigeon-toed). Distribute your weight equally between both feet, and on each foot feel the base of the big and little toes and both sides of the heel pressing down. Extend your bodyweight up from these points.

❷ Lift your toes, splay them, hold, then replace on the floor one by one, trying to maintain a gap between each toe.

❸ Feel your toes and the four parts of each foot anchored to the floor. To check this solidity, sway forward and back and from side to side until you find a point just forward from your heels at which you gain an effortless energy lift.

20 Animating the joints

❶ Stand with feet hip-width apart, establishing a base as on page 29. Lift up through your ankles, drawing energy up the back of the knees and thighs.

❷ Pull up through both hips, tucking your pelvis slightly up and under, lower back lengthening. Draw the abdomen in and up as you extend through your torso equally on both sides, opening your chest and relaxing your shoulders away from your ears. Stretch your arms down, forearms drawing in.

❸ Tuck your chin toward your throat, parallel to the floor. Imagine a string at the crown of your head pulling you toward the ceiling. Hold for 30 seconds or more, feeling the extension from ankles to crown, and vital energy coursing up your spine.

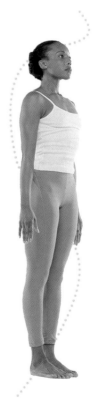

21 For neck and shoulders

❶ Exhaling, take your chin down to your throat, compressing the thyroid. Inhaling, pivot your head to point your chin at the ceiling. Exhale back to center.

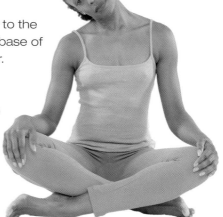

❷ On an exhalation, drop the left ear to the left shoulder. Start the stretch in the base of your spine and extend it up and over. Inhale to center; repeat to the right.

❸ Exhale, tuck your chin in, parallel to the floor, feel a lift up the back of the skull. Inhale and take your chin forward. Exhale to center.

❹ Inhaling, pivot your head to look left. Exhale and look behind. Inhale back to center, and exhale. Repeat to the right.

22 Vigor for the legs

❶ Sit with legs outstretched, arms by your sides, palms pressing down by your hips, fingers pointing forward. Pivot forward from the hips and pull out excess flesh from beneath your sitting bones. Come back to center.

❷ Exhaling, lengthen through the back of your thighs, calves, and heels, pushing the energy through both edges of the foot and drawing your toes toward your knees.

❸ Inhaling, sit tall, pulling out of your pelvis and stretching each side equally from hips to underarms. Open your chest, pull your chin toward your throat, and feel energy rising up the back of your skull to your crown. Hold for 30 seconds.

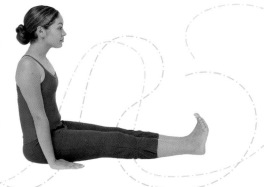

23 Firing up the lower back

❶ Stand in Tadasana (page 30). Inhaling, extend your arms overhead. Hold for a couple of breath cycles, then, exhaling, hinge forward from the hips.

❷ Fold your arms and allow them to hang loosely or plant your palms either side of the feet, fingers forward, base of the palms by your heels.

❸ Relax into the pose, releasing head and shoulders, and moving your hips forward until your weight descends through the balls of your feet. Keep your feet active.

❹ Hold for 30 seconds or more. With each exhalation, let gravity lengthen the spine away from the hips and release the back of the legs. Come up slowly on an inhalation, head last.

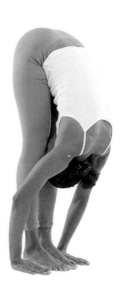

24 Numb bum buster

❶ Lying on your back, bring your knees toward your chest. Clasp your upper shins with both hands and with each exhalation, bring your knees further in to massage your abdomen. Lift your head to your knees to stretch the whole spine. Hold for up to 30 seconds.

❷ It can be soothing to rock in this position. Place your head down. Using your hands, and co-ordinating with your breathing, slowly take your knees out and around in a circle, first clockwise, then anticlockwise, sensing every part of the back of the pelvis make contact with the floor. Release legs to the floor.

25 Spine energizer

❶ Lie on your back with knees bent, feet flat on the floor. Spread your arms out, shoulders and back of the hands flat to the mat.

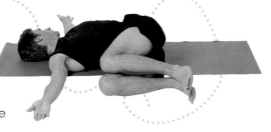

❷ Roll on to your left side, stacking knees and ankles, and place your right palm on your left palm. Turn your head to gaze along the line of your arm.

❸ Inhaling, lift your right arm to the ceiling; exhaling, return it to its original position on the floor.

❹ Hold for 30 seconds or more, knees and ankles still stacked and resting on the floor. Inhale into areas of stiffness, and with each exhalation try to take both shoulders nearer the floor. Repeat to the other side.

26 After long periods of sitting

❶ Sit in Dandasana (page 32). Bend your right leg and place the foot near the right buttock. Extend the straight leg, toes pointing up.

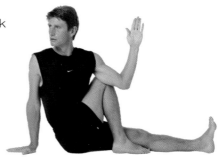

❷ Exhale and, keeping your back straight and hips forward, twist your torso to the right. If you can, take your left shoulder in front of your right knee, elbow bent, palm facing right. If not, grasp the knee. Keep the bent knee upright.

❸ Extend the spine, and plant the right palm behind your right hip. Turn to look as far behind as possible. Hold for 30 seconds, with each inhalation extending the spine and rotating further. Keep rooting both hips equally and extend the outstretched leg. Inhale back to center. Repeat to the other side.

27 After long periods of standing

❶ Kneel on the mat, knees together, feet and ankles touching, buttocks on your heels.

❷ Lengthen your spine, drawing out of both hips equally and opening the chest, shoulders away from ears. Rest your hands on your knees. Hold for 30 seconds or more, breathing space into the lower legs and flattening out sore feet and ankles.

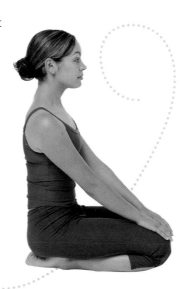

❸ As a variation, kneel up and tuck your toes under, big toes touching. Sit back on your heels so your bodyweight compresses your toes. Hold for just longer than you can bear, breathing into any areas that may hurt.

28 Hand and wrist reviver

❶ Sitting comfortably upright, bring palms and fingers together in front of your chest. Press your thumbs lightly into your sternum as you inhale, opening your chest. Hold for a few breath cycles, focusing on each digit in turn. Then take your palms up to touch thumbs between your eyes. Hold for a few breath cycles.

❷ Take your arms behind your back and place your palms together at your lower back, fingers pointing down. Turn your hands in and up, palms and fingers still touching, to form reverse prayer position. Open your chest and work your elbows to manoeuvre your palms together, taking them up between your shoulder blades. Hold, inhaling into the tension, for a few breath cycles. If impossible, simply grasp opposite elbows behind your back.

Pose > Adho mukha svanasana
Level > beginner
Good for > exercising the muscles of the arms and shoulders

29 Revitalizing shoulders

❶ Start on hands and knees, hips and
legs, shoulders and arms creating
right angles. Turn your toes
under your feet.

❷ Exhaling, press back on
your palms to lift your hips
high and bend your knees.
Focus on pressing your
sitting bones to the ceiling
and lengthening the back.

❸ Relax your neck and head, draw out of the shoulders,
and widen the shoulder blades. Try to straighten your legs,
pressing your heels toward the ground. Hold for 30 seconds
or more, simultaneously extending the legs into the heels, the
arms out of the shoulders, and the sitting bones pointing up
toward the ceiling.

Pose > Urdhva mukha svanasana
Level > intermediate
Good for > boosting circulation and exercising the arms and shoulders

30 Reviving the upper-body

❶ Lying prone with legs outstretched and touching, forehead on the floor and arms by your sides, bend your elbows and take your palms beneath your shoulders, fingers forward, elbows pressing in.

❷ Inhaling, turn your toes under and lift your body off the floor like a plank. Pressing down through hands and toes, raise your chest and head, chin pointing up toward the ceiling.

❸ Hold for 30 seconds, opening your chest, releasing your shoulders from your ears, and feeling energy running down your strong, stable arms. Do not compress your lower back.

31 Easing rounded shoulders

❶ Kneel on the mat, legs forming a right angle with the floor, tops of the feet pressing down. Extend the spine, making a straight line from knees through hips, shoulders, and neck.

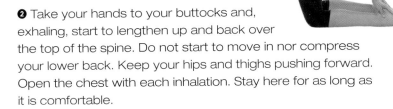

❷ Take your hands to your buttocks and, exhaling, start to lengthen up and back over the top of the spine. Do not start to move in nor compress your lower back. Keep your hips and thighs pushing forward. Open the chest with each inhalation. Stay here for as long as it is comfortable.

❸ Take back one, then the other hand to cup each heel. Drop your head to look behind, focusing on the exhilarating stretch in the throat and armpits. Keep your hips forward (retain the right angle with the floor), and stretch up from your wrists. Hold for 30 seconds; inhale back upright.

32 For stamina

❶ Lie prone, forehead on the ground, legs stretched out behind. Exhaling, lengthen your legs away from your lower back and open your chest into the floor.

❷ Inhaling, bend your legs at the knees. On the next exhalation, reach back and grab your ankles.

❸ Keeping your hips and groin pressing down, inhale and raise your chest, simultaneously lifting your legs up and away so the thighs rise. Look forward.

❹ Hold for up to 20 seconds, extending the front of the body and front of the thighs equally, pivoting from the center. Lower your legs carefully to the floor on an exhalation.

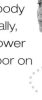

33 Digestive energy-raiser

❶ Lie prone, forehead on the ground and legs stretched out behind, feet together, toes pointing away. Plant your hands beneath your shoulders, fixing palms and fingers to the ground, elbows in. Exhaling, extend your legs back and spine forward, lengthening the lower back.

❷ Inhaling, lift the upper body forward and up. Do not press on the arms to achieve a stretch, and do not compress the lower back. Drop the shoulders, broaden the chest, and point your chin up.

❸ Hold for up to 30 seconds, focusing on the chest opening and shoulders dropping, straightening the arms if desired. Exhaling, unroll down slowly.

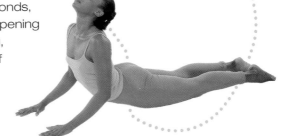

34 Stoking digestive fire

❶ Sit in Vajrasana (page 37). Kneel up and step your left leg forward, knee over ankle to create a right angle. Rest your palms on your front knee.

❷ Exhaling, take your trunk and front leg forward without moving the foot so your back leg stretches into a lunge. Hold for a few breath cycles, breathing into the extended back thigh and stabilizing the upper body over the front heel.

❸ Inhaling, stretch your arms forward and up, extending out of the hips equally on both sides and releasing the shoulders down. On the next inhalation, stretch up and back to avoid compressing the lower spine. Open the chest and take the head back, chin pointing up. Hold for up to 30 seconds. Inhale to come up; repeat to the other side.

Pose > Mukha svanasana sequence
Level > advanced
Good for > increasing stamina, toning, cardiovascular workout

35 Total invigoration workout

❶ Start on hands and knees. Turn your toes under. Exhaling, lift the hips high and press back with the arms into Adho Mukha Svanasana (page 39). Relax your neck. Press heels toward the ground and buttocks to the ceiling while lifting out of the shoulders.

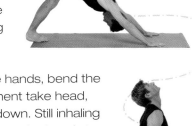

❷ Inhaling, press forward onto the hands, bend the elbows and in one flowing movement take head, shoulders, and hips forward and down. Still inhaling and keeping the move fluid, press on the hands to arch the upper body into Urdhva Mukha Svanasana (page 40).

❸ Exhaling, press on the hands and take the hips back up into Adho Mukha Svanasana. Move between the 2 poses 3 or 5 times in a fluid sequence, then sink your hips back onto your heels and rest in Balasana (page 59).

36 Posture boost

❶ Stand in Tadasana (page 30), feet hip-width apart. Pull up from a secure base, stacking knees, hips, and shoulders.

❷ Bring your palms together in prayer position at the buttocks (page 38, step 2). Turn them in and up, sliding your hands between your shoulder blades without thumbs separating. Alternatively, grasp opposite elbows.

❸ Step your feet 3ft apart, right foot out 90°, left in 60°. Turn the shoulders and hips right and square. Inhaling, lift the chest and chin; look up.

❹ Exhaling, pivot forward from the hips, upper body out and down toward the front leg, neck relaxed. Hold for 30 seconds, breathing space into the back of the legs and rooting through both feet to maintain balance. Inhale up. Repeat to the left.

Refreshing
the senses

Yoga massages the senses with spot-focus
exercises and with meditations that help
you see the world afresh.

37 Eye energizer

❶ Sit comfortably upright on the floor, hands resting on knees or thighs. Place a nightlight on a low table, level with your eyes. Settle yourself by watching your breathing for a moment, then focus your gaze on the tip of the flame, at the point at which its form and color disappear.

❷ Keep your gaze steady and uninterrupted on the flame for up to 1 minute, trying not to blink. Then close your eyes and see the flame in your mind's eye.

❸ When the image has faded, open your eyes, and repeat the gaze. Work for up to 3 minutes, using the image of the flame to cleanse your mind of other thoughts.

38 Energy eyebath

❶ Standing in Tadasana (page 30), rub your palms together to generate heat and energy. Then press the center of each palm with the opposite thumb 3 times to stimulate energy points.

❷ Cup your palms gently over your eyes so it is completely dark. Don't press on your eyeballs. Look into the darkness, focusing on the area between your eyebrows, the third eye. Take your hands away, opening your eyes.

❸ Keeping your head completely still, look left, hold, then right. Look to the floor, then the ceiling. Try not to blink. Look up to the left and down to the right, then up to the right and down to the left. Finally, make a large, slow circle with your eyes, as if following the hands round a clockface. Work in both directions.

39 Palate awakener

❶ Look at the food before you as if for the first time. Note its colors, temperature, textures, and the complex blend of aromas it emits.

❷ Close your eyes as you place a morsel in your mouth. Pause before chewing, and let the flavors activate tastebuds at various points on your tongue. Do nothing else: do not talk, think, or become distracted.

❸ Then, as you chew, activate the muscles in your jaw and neck, sense the connections between hand and brain as you lift your fork, feel your teeth coming together. Slow down to appreciate each mouthful in the moment.

40 Ear reviver

❶ Sit in a comfortable upright position, hands resting on thighs or knees. Close your eyes and watch your breathing, clearing your mind as the breath moves in and out.

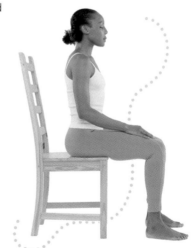

❷ Focus on sounds in the room. What can you hear with your left ear? What can you hear with your right? What sounds can you hear in front and behind you?

❸ Now listen outside the room. What can you hear immediately beyond you; what sounds are in the building? What can you hear outdoors? Try to extend your hearing beyond the traffic and birdsong, wind, and rustling of trees to sense the world spinning.

Pose > Setu bandha sarvangasana
Level > beginner
Good for > instant radiance, refreshing the face with oxygenated blood

41 Skin freshener

❶ Lie on your back, bend your knees, and place your feet flat on the floor, hip-width apart, close to your buttocks. Make sure the outside edges are parallel. Keep your arms close by your side.

❷ Inhaling, raise your hips, pressing the back of your arms and tops of shoulders down. Hold for up to 1 minute, keeping the hips and thighs lifting, abdomen tucked in and up, and grounding down through your heels. With each inhalation open your chest; keep it opening as you exhale, pressing down through your shoulders. Slowly exhale to the floor vertebra by vertebra.

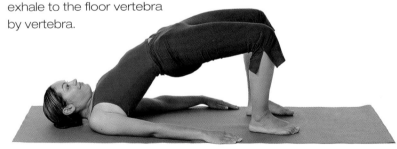

42 Instant facelift

Found in the web of skin between thumb and index finger, "Chinese Acupoint Large Intestine 4" stimulates a flow of energy to the upper body that results in a radiant complexion. Apply gentle pressure to the spot using the thumb and first finger of the opposite hand for 30 seconds. Repeat on the other hand.

43 Zesty scents

Burn incense and essential oils to invigorate your space: choose sandalwood for spiritual energy, peppermint for mind revival, and ginger to enliven the body.

44 Restoring energy vibes

To get the most out of yoga, engage all your senses and focus in the present. Chime cymbals to cleanse the space. Place energy-raising gels in yellow, orange, and red tones over windows to suffuse the room with renewing light. Sip energy-raising herbal teas: fennel is celebrated as a tonic for restoring the power of youth to a jaded palate, and raising agni, the body's digestive fire. Peppermint has been shown in Japanese studies to sharpen mental performance.

45 Energy superfoods

Choose quick-fix energy foods to supplement revitalizing yoga postures. Ayurvedic practitioners advise adding fresh ginger root and lime juice to food to kindle "agni," the fire that counters a sluggish digestion; and prescribe dates for early morning energy, plus mango juice for sheer vitality.

46 Sensory meditation

❶ Start sitting comfortably upright. Examine an object of beauty—a statue of Buddha, a flower, an icon—to fix it in your memory in three dimensions, turning it around to view it from every angle. While doing so, think not only about its physical form, but the qualities it embodies: perhaps compassion, love, serenity.

❷ Close your eyes and visualize the image appearing in an intense light between and in front of your eyebrows. Focus your mind on its form and qualities; feel its essence with every sense. When your mind starts to drift, redirect it to the object. Work for 3 minutes.

47 Sensing courage

❶ Sit in Vajrasana (page 37), extending your spine from sitting bones to crown.

❷ Leaning back, place your hands behind your toes. Inhaling, lift your thighs to take your pelvis to the ceiling. Carefully take the head back to look behind.

❸ Hold for 30 seconds, feeling an opening through your armpits and a bold broadening of the chest. Let the extension in the neck energize your sense organs. Exhale back to Vajrasana, then rest forward in Balasana (page 59).

Recharging
the system

Use the exercises that follow to bring refreshment to stale ways of thinking that stop you from being fully alive, and to replenish your take on the world with a new input of creativity.

48 Replenishing

❶ Sit in Dandasana (page 32). Take your arms overhead on an inhalation. Stretch equally on both sides.

❷ Exhaling, hinge forward from the hips. Place your hands on your calves, ankles, or toes, and open the chest as you bend forward, extending from the lower back and looking forward. Do not round the back.

❸ With each exhalation, extend a little further, till the abdomen, chest, and finally the forehead come to rest on the legs. Place your hands on or beyond the feet. Rest here for up to 1 minute, keeping the navel moving forward with each out-breath, and breathing into tension at the back of the legs. Inhale to come up.

49 Refocusing thoughts

❶ Kneel with your buttocks on your heels. Bend forward, letting your chest relax fully onto both thighs before taking your forehead or crown of the head to rest on the floor. Let your arms lie quietly beside your body, hands by your feet.

❷ Simply breathe in the pose for 1 minute or more, feeling your lower back expand with each inhalation and letting every part of you go with the exhalation. Let your torso melt into your thighs.

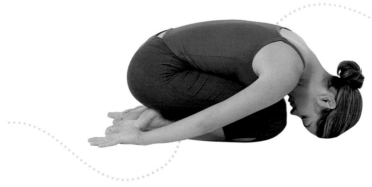

50 Repairing frayed nerves

❶ Stand in Tadasana (page 30). Stabilize your weight on your left leg. Bend your right leg, take the foot to the buttock, and clasp it with your right hand.

❷ With shoulders and hips square, torso extending on both sides, exhale and stretch your left arm overhead, palm forward.

❸ Exhaling, tilt your body forward from your hips, left arm moving forward and up. Stretch back your right arm to draw the foot back and up.

❹ Hold for up to 30 seconds, hips square, extending the spine and right leg without compressing the lower back. Feel the energy strung between the back leg pulling back and torso pulling forward. Repeat on the other side.

51 Reviving a jaded outlook

❶ Stand in Tadasana (page 30). Inhaling, jump or step the feet 3–4ft apart. Pull up from ankles to hips. Center your pelvis, abdomen up and in, square your shoulders, and lengthen the spine to the crown. Extend your arms parallel to the floor, palms down, stretching through thumbs and little fingers.

❷ Turn your left foot out 90°, right foot in 60°. Inhaling, raise your right arm and extend your torso left, bringing your left hand to your calf, ankle, or the floor. Reach to the ceiling with your upper arm, drawing your fingertips up. Look at your top thumb.

❸ Hold for 30–60 seconds. With each inhalation, extend your arms, and lengthen from the base of the spine to the crown. Anchor the back foot and pull the buttocks together. Inhale to come up. Repeat to the other side.

52 Power-builder

❶ Stand in Tadasana (page 30). Inhaling, step the feet 3–4ft apart. Center your pelvis, pull abdomen up and in, square your shoulders, and lengthen the spine to the crown. Extend the arms parallel to the floor, palms down, stretching through the fingers.

❷ Turn your left foot out 90°, right foot in 45°. Exhaling, bend your left knee over the heel, thigh parallel to the floor. Sink your pelvis, weight equal in both thighs. Look along your left arm.

❸ Hold for 30–60 seconds. With each inhalation, extend the spine and lengthen the arms and chest, shoulderblades broadening. Keep your back leg strong, anchoring the outer edge of the foot, buttocks pulling toward each other. Inhale to straighten the bent leg. Repeat to the other side.

53 Increasing dynamism

❶ Follow step 1 of Virabhadrasana (page 62).

❷ Turn your left foot out 90° and pivot your right foot in so your right hip faces forward. Bend your front knee over the ankle, thigh parallel to the floor, torso square.

❸ Inhaling, take your arms overhead, bringing the palms together in prayer position. Look at your palms, or gently drop your head back. Hold for 30–60 seconds. With each inhalation, stretch up from the firm anchor of your pelvis. Feel your feet rooted to the floor, your back leg anchored. Inhale to come up, and repeat to the other side.

54 When stress drains you

❶ Sit in Vajrasana (page 37). Drop your chest on to your thighs. On an exhalation, place the crown of your head on the floor in front of your knees.

❷ Place your elbows by your ears, resting your palms on the floor. Exhaling, lift your buttocks to take your hips up in a straight line over your knees.

❸ Stretch your arms back to clasp your heels. Hold for 30–60 seconds without collapsing the inner circle created between chest and thighs. Relax back in Balasana (page 59) by taking your buttocks to your heels without lifting your head. Inhale to come up.

55 Confidence-booster

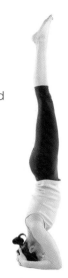

❶ Kneeling, grasp opposite elbows and place them on the floor. Open out your forearms to form a triangle, and interlace your fingers. Place them perpendicular to the floor, little fingers down.

❷ Place the crown down, cradling the back of your head in the cup of your fingers. Straighten your legs and walk in until your spine is straight, hips over shoulders. Practice until you feel stable.

❸ Bend your knees, press your forearms down, and, exhaling, lift your legs until your knees align over your shoulders and hips. Take a few breaths, spine perpendicular, shoulderblades pulling in. Look ahead.

❹ Exhaling, straighten your legs, squeezing the thighs in and up. On each inhalation, lift through the shoulders and pull the abdomen in and up. Hold for 3 minutes. Descend slowly. Keep your head down for 30 seconds.

56 Breathing for energy

❶ Sit comfortably upright, either on the floor with legs crossed and back straight, or on an upright chair, feet flat on the ground. Place your hands low over your abdomen, with your fingertips touching.

❷ As you breathe in, bypass your chest and feel the air drop toward the abdomen, causing your fingertips to draw away from each other.

❸ As you exhale, imagine the breath leaving your abdomen little by little from the top down and notice your fingertips touch again. Work for 3–4 minutes, watching your breath lengthen and deepen.

57 Hearing energy flow

❶ Sit comfortably upright, hands resting on either your knees or thighs. Close your eyes and focus on your securely planted sitting bones and regular breathing.

❷ Inhale through both nostrils, letting the breath drop to your abdomen. Feel your diaphragm sink, abdomen expand, and ribcage widen.

❸ On the exhalation, contract your throat as if starting to hum, and expel air gradually from the top down, feeling a whispering "haaa" in your throat. Take a regular breath, if required, before starting the next cycle.

❹ Repeat for 3–5 minutes, keeping the cycles smooth, steady, and rhythmic, and letting the in-breath come naturally. Once you are used to the rustling "haaaa" sound on the exhalation, start to feel it on the inhalation too.

58 Rediscovering fun

❶ Sit comfortably upright, hands resting on knees or thighs. Close your eyes and watch your regular breathing for a few cycles, feeling your breath deepen and lengthen.

❷ Breathe in through both nostrils. Open your mouth slightly and let the exhalation vibrate through loose, open lips to make a continuous hum. Don't worry if this makes you laugh at first.

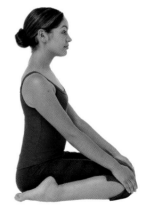

❸ Repeat the inhalation and humming exhalation up to 7 times, keeping the sound smooth and uninterrupted, and feeling the vibration on your lips, palate, back of the throat, and eventually from the base of the spine to the crown of your head.

59 Energy breath

❶ Sit comfortably upright. Fold your right first and middle fingers into your palm. Take your hand to your nose. Place the ring and little fingers on your left nostril, the thumb on your right nostril. Join the left thumb and first finger—Vishnu mudra.

❷ Close your eyes. Inhale through both nostrils, block your left nostril with ring and little fingers, and exhale through your right nostril. Inhale though your right nostril, envisaging activating energy.

❸ At the top of the inhalation, block your right nostril with the thumb, and exhale through your left nostril. Inhale through your left nostril, feeling a cooling detoxifying. This is 1 cycle. Repeat up to 7 cycles. Finish on an exhalation from the right nostril, then go back to inhaling through both nostrils.

60 Energy chant

The sound Om (pronounced AUM) is said to be the essence of everything—the utterance that brought forth the universe. As such, it is energy incarnate, and to chant it brings you into harmony with the energy of the cosmos. Chant sitting comfortably upright: inhale deeply, and start the utterance on the out-breath, resonating the "AAA" in the abdomen, "OOO" in the throat, and "MMM" at the palate with mouth closed, opening the lips to let the final sound trail out to merge imperceptibly with the energy of the universe.

61 Power mantra

Chanting was recommended by ancient Indian sages to generate harmony, concentration, and creative power. The mantra Som (pronounced like "home") imparts energy and vitality and has a strengthening and rejuvenating effect. Repeat it out loud at first, then as it feels comfortable, repeat silently when in need of an energy-boost.

Spirit-raising

With yoga you can learn to perceive prana, life's energy force, running into and through you as your limbs, your spine, and the crown of your head experience a magical tingling and shaking.

62 Feeling the force

❶ Stand with your back 1ft in front of a wall. Bend your knees and press your spine against the wall, from your pelvis to head, taking your lower back and back of the neck toward the support.

❷ Look down without moving your head, and sink until you see your knees. Press the back of your arms and hands into the wall. Hold for up to 3 minutes, with each out-breath increasing contact.

❸ Stand away from the wall in Tadasana (page 30), feet hip-width apart or together, knees slightly bent. Take your arms away from your body, as if holding oranges beneath your armpits, fingers flexed out. Hold, breathing, for 1 minute or more, sensing tingling in your fingers and along your spine.

63 Energy-shifting

To perceive how different yoga poses cause energy to shift around the body, go into Savasana (page 10) or Balasana (page 59) between postures and feel which areas feel invigorated or pulsate with new life.

64 Breathing life into the hara

When lying in Savasana (page 10), on an in-breath imagine sucking energy into the body though the toes and fingertips. Direct it up your legs, up your arms, and down your spine to ignite the energy reservoir situated below your navel, known as the hara in Traditional Chinese and Japanese Medicine. When you exhale, take energy from this vital pool and let it suffuse every part of the body.

65 Energy pause

❶ Sit comfortably upright, hands resting on knees or thighs. Close your eyes and focus on your regular breathing.

❷ Inhale to a count of 3. Pause, holding for 3, then exhale for 3. This is one cycle. Take a regular breath, if necessary. Repeat 3, 5, or 7 cycles. Work with this for some weeks.

❸ Now start to lengthen the out-breath. Inhale for 3, pause for 3, and exhale to the count of 6. Take a regular breath, if necessary. As you pause, retaining the breath, do not let the shoulders rise, but feel a sense of profound clarity. On the exhalation, let calmness envelop you. Work for 3–5 minutes.

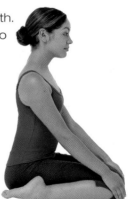

66 Energizing the heart center 1

❶ Sit in Vajrasana (page 37), then come up to kneeling, hips centered over knees, shoulders squared over the hips, feet pressing down, and toes pointing away.

❷ Inhaling, raise the arms overhead, palms forward, and hold for a few breath cycles, releasing the shoulders away from the ears and keeping the extension equal on both sides of the body.

❸ On another inhalation, take your arms back, extending the upper back without compressing the lower back. Gently take your head back, pointing your chin up. Work for up to 30 seconds, feeling an opening and energizing of the chest. Come up on an inhalation.

67 Energizing the heart center 2

❶ Standing in Tadasana (page 30) with feet hip-width apart, inhale and raise your arms overhead, palms forward. Release your shoulders downward and make sure your torso is square and extending equally on both sides.

❷ Root down through your hips, knees, and heels, then inhaling, slowly take your arms and upper spine back. Draw up and out of your pelvis to avoid compressing the lower back. Gently drop your head back, ears in line with your arms, looking forward and up.

❸ Hold for 20–30 seconds, pushing your hips forward slightly, rooting down, and opening the chest over the arch of the spine. Come up on an inhalation.

68 Color visualization

Meditate on a color to get heart energy circulating. The heart chakra, anahata, resonates to a shade of green: imagine the color suffusing your heart region with each inhalation as you sit to meditate or breathe, and when working on chest-expanding postures.

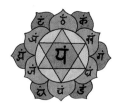

69 Releasing throat energy

Energy that gets stuck in the throat area can prevent good communication and self-expression. Release it by envisaging a purplish-blue light enveloping the throat chakra, vishuddha, during meditation or breathing exercises, or while taking the head back in yoga postures.

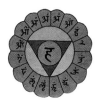

70 Blasting the chakras

❶ Lie on your back, legs outstretched, arms by your side. Bend your knees, placing your feet near your buttocks, hip-width apart, outer edges parallel.

❷ Stretch your arms up, bend the elbows, and insert your hands, palms down, beneath the top of each shoulder, fingers toward the feet. Work here until you can press down comfortably and firmly.

❸ Inhaling, press into the palms and soles to raise the body into an arch, head dropping to look back, pelvis the highest point. Hold for 20–30 seconds, pressing firmly out of the shoulders. Do not compress the lower back, and keep the chest opening through the armpits with each inhalation. Descend slowly, exhaling.

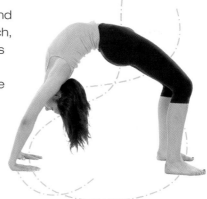

71 Rousing kundalini

❶ Sit in Dandasana (page 32). Bend your left leg and place the heel near the right buttock, toes pointing away. Bend your right leg over the left leg, ankle by the knee, toes pointing left to make a diagonal line with your left heel and toes.

❷ Exhale and, keeping your back straight, hips forward, and top knee upright, twist right to take your left tricep back against your right knee and calf. Extend the arm, gently resting the left hand on your right foot.

72 Conserving raised energy

❶ From Sarvangasana (page 85), lower your extended legs to the ground behind your head. Keep the spine extending from the back of the neck up to the pelvis, and rest your feet on tiptoes, heels stretching away.

❷ Stretch your arms along the floor behind you, interlocking fingers if desired. Fix your gaze on your navel, inhaling deep in the abdomen. Hold for 3 minutes or more. Curl down slowly, vertebra by vertebra, on an exhalation.

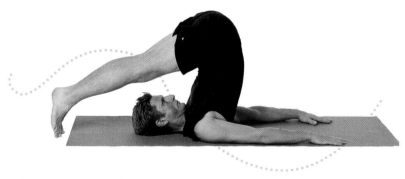

73 Trapping energy

❶ From Halasana (page 80), bend your knees and draw them toward your shoulders, blocking your ears. Close your eyes and focus on your breath.

❷ Fold your arms around the back of your knees, clasping opposite forearms. Switch off from the world for 30 seconds or more. Release the arms and curl down slowly, vertebra by vertebra, on an exhalation.

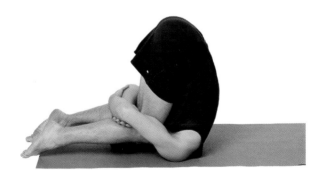

74 The energy of inner peace

Recognize that energy comes from within—from being the best possible person you can. The law of karma, followed by millions of Hindus, Buddhists, and Jains the world over, states that if you behave in a kind and compassionate way, responding with love, patience, and understanding to those around you, and seeking to find peace through meditation, yoga, and seeing the divine aspect of everything, then positive energy rebounds on you and reveals itself in every part of you, from your posture and zest for life to the radiance of your skin.

Everyday energizers

Yoga offers an energy blast wherever you are, whatever the situation, and at any time of day or night.

75 Wake-up call

❶ Stand in Tadasana (page 30), feet together. Find a stable base between the heels and balls of the feet, and inhale energy up through your ankles, knees, and thighs.

❷ Keep energy rising through your pelvis, tilting it forward slightly, and pull your abdomen back. Keep extending as you inhale, feeling energy expand your chest.

❸ Lift the back of the skull away from the neck, chin in, shoulders released from ears. Inhale, raise arms overhead, forearms toward each other, feeling energy flow from fingertips to ankles.

❹ Inhaling, bend left, arms still extending. Hold for 20–30 seconds, stretching both sides. Inhale to center; repeat to the right. Exhale the arms down.

76 Relieving morning tiredness

❶ Lie on your back, knees bent. Press your elbows into the floor, exhale, and lift your legs and torso. Place your hands on your lower back on either side of the spine, fingers up. Exhaling, press on your arms and take your body up until your legs are at 45°. Stay here until you feel confident.

❷ Inch your hands down toward your shoulderblades. Exhaling, extend your legs to form a straight line from shoulders to heels, chest near the chin, elbows coming together. Hold for 3 minutes or more. Look at your navel, lifting your torso and legs, shoulders stable and chest broad.

❸ Exhaling, lower down vertebra by vertebra, legs at an angle, outstretched arms like brakes. When the legs reach 90°, bend them to the floor.

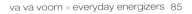

77 AM energy blast

❶ Stand in Tadasana (page 30), palms in prayer position.

❷ Inhaling, stretch your arms overhead and back, looking behind.

❸ Exhaling, bend forward from the hips into Uttanasana (page 11). Plant your palms by your feet.

❹ Inhaling, take your left leg back in a lunge, right heel flat. Bring your chest and chin up.

❺ Take the right leg back behind you and hold yourself on hands and feet like an angled plank; look forward.

❻ Exhaling, relax back onto bent knees, arms forward.

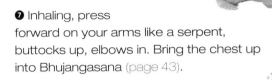

❼ Inhaling, press
forward on your arms like a serpent,
buttocks up, elbows in. Bring the chest up
into Bhujangasana (page 43).

❽ Exhaling, push your hips up into
Adho Mukha Svanasana (page 39).

❾ Inhaling, step your right leg forward in
a lunge, look up, as step 4.

❿ Exhaling, bring your
back leg forward and raise
your buttocks, as step 3.

⓫ Inhaling, come to standing, taking your arms
overhead and back, as step 2.

78 Post-prandial energizer

❶ Lie on your front, legs outstretched and touching, arms by your side (palms up), forehead on the floor. Exhaling, stretch your legs away from your spine.

❷ Imagine your thighs are heavy: with legs straight, inhale and raise both calves, as if trying to place your soles on the ceiling. Simultaneously lift your head, chest, and arms (parallel to the floor, palms facing). Look forward and up.

❸ Hold for a few breath cycles, keeping feet and head at the same level. Lower with control on an exhalation.

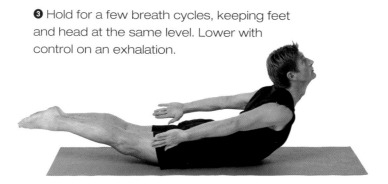

79 After-lunch slump

❶ Sit in Dandasana (page 32). Leaning back slightly, lift the legs, knees bent, and raise the arms parallel to the floor, palms facing each other. Keep knees and feet aligned with the shoulders, and breathe. Remain here until you feel stable.

❷ Extend the legs, pushing through the heels, and stretch through the fingertips. Lift or lower the back and legs until both tilt at the same angle and the head and feet align.

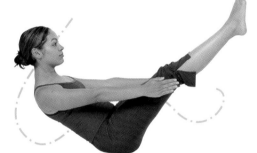

❸ Hold for up to 20 seconds, steadying your breath, and lifting the chest and spine. Exhale back to Dandasana.

80 Mid-afternoon pick-me-up

❶ Stand in Tadasana (page 30). Inhaling, jump or step the feet 3–4 ft apart. Turn the right foot out 90°, left foot in slightly. Extend your arms, palms down.

❷ Bend your right knee; place your right hand on the floor in front of your toes. Straighten your right leg, slowly raising the left leg.

❸ Keeping the right leg aligned hip over ankle and left leg straight, pelvis opening, raise your ribs and left arm to align with the lower arm. Carefully look up. Hold for 20 seconds or more, breathing stability into the grounded foot and stretching between both hands, and between raised foot and crown of the head. Repeat to the left.

81 When you simply can't stop

Use this walking meditation to refocus your energies during a busy day. As you start walking, switch off your thoughts and tune into your breathing; watch how the in- and out-breaths fall in time with your pace. Start to slow your pace, becoming aware of your feet lifting and being replaced on the ground. Focus on your breathing, inhaling for two paces and exhaling for two paces. Feel your thoughts steady with your pace until you find yourself moving in meditation.

82 Energy on the go

When you are active, be mindful of the center of your energy, feeling every movement start from the hara energy reservoir low in your abdomen. When cycling, jogging, walking, or swimming, gather yourself from this point and direct energy out around your body to increase your sense of spirit, improve your posture, and so make every movement more energy-efficient.

83 Evening energy wind-down

❶ Stand in Tadasana (page 30), palms in prayer position. Inhaling, raise your arms overhead and slightly back.

❷ Exhaling, bend forward into Uttanasana (page 11), palms planted by your feet.

❸ Inhaling, take the right leg back in a lunge, knee up. Lift your torso and look forward, palms in prayer position. Inhaling, extend your arms to the sides, straighten the legs, then turn right.

❹ Turn to front, and place the right knee down. Lunge forward, left knee over the foot. Inhaling, raise your arms into Anjaneyasana (page 44).

❺ Come down to hands and knees, with the next in-breath, push your hips up into Adho Mukha Svanasana (page 39).

❻ Bend your arms, lowering your shoulders, and, inhaling, push forward and up into Urdhva Mukha Svanasana (page 40). Exhaling, press back into Adho Mukha Svanasana. Relax onto bent knees, arms forward.

❼ Come to kneeling, legs perpendicular, hands in prayer position. Inhaling, raise hands and chin up and back in Nagasana (page 75).

❽ Come back to hands and knees. Exhaling, push into Adho Mukha Svanasana. Bend your arms and, inhaling, push into Urdhva Mukha Svanasana. Exhaling, press back into Adho Mukha Svanasana.

❾ Look to your hands, inhale, and jump your feet between them into Uttanasana.

❿ Inhale to standing, raising your arms overhead and back. Exhaling, bring your hands back to prayer position. Repeat the steps, leading with the other leg; turn left in step 4.

84 Bedtime energy calming

Massage is a key Ayurvedic adjunct to yoga, a way of
ensuring that life's energy, prana, flows through the body's
subtle energy channels as it should. Like yoga postures,
massage works on 107 marma points, or energy junctions,
and seven energy centers, chakras, situated on the nadi
channels running through the body. Before bed each night
after your yoga wind-down, massage the soles and tops of
the feet and your scalp with warmed sesame oil, using firm,
smooth, rhythmic strokes. By morning, body and face will
appear rested and radiant.

Anywhere lethargy zappers

Tiredness, listlessness, and nervous exhaustion can strike anywhere—in a meeting, on the road, even in bed—zapping your zest for life and ability to function at your peak. Let these exercises renew your energy.

85 At the wheel

❶ Circle your hands from the wrists, without moving your arms, outward, then inward.

❷ Interlace your fingers and push your arms forward, pressing out through the wrists. Raise the interlinked arms overhead, if possible, maintaining the push through the wrists. Repeat, this time placing the other first finger forward when interlinking hands.

❸ Pivot forward to bend your left arm behind your back, elbow close in. Press the back of the palm up between the shoulder blades. Extend the other arm overhead, bend the elbow, and take the hand, palm inward, down between the shoulder blades. Try to grasp the lower hand, or simply inch the hands toward each other. Repeat on the other arm.

86 On the train or plane

❶ Sit upright, soles flat on the floor. Lift your toes, keeping the rest of the feet down. Extend the toes wide, little toes stretching away from big toes. Replace your big toes, keeping the other toes up. Then lift the big toes, other toes down.

❷ Raise one knee to lift the foot. Pull your toes strongly toward your knee; hold for a few breath cycles. Point your toes away, holding an intense stretch through the top of the foot. Repeat on the other foot.

❸ With knee still lifted, circle your feet from the ankles without moving the lower leg: describe a circle the size of a plate with your big toe. Work in both directions, then repeat on the other foot.

87 Before an interview

❶ Sit in Dandasana (page 32). Bend the right leg, taking the foot against the left thigh near the groin.

❷ Bend the left leg. Support beneath the foot with both hands and place it on the right thigh, outer edge by the groin, sole up—Half-lotus Pose. Practice on both legs before bringing the right foot over the left knee on to the left thigh, outer edge near the groin, sole up—Lotus Pose.

❸ Breathe into areas of pain and release tension with each out-breath. Inhale the spine upward. Watch your breathing, gradually lengthening the out-breath (to a count of 5 or 7).

❹ Work for 3–5 minutes, relinquishing residual tension, and feeling each inhalation bring new confidence. Exhale to uncurl each leg.

88 At your desk

❶ Center your shoulders over your hips and bring your chin in toward your throat, thereby extending the back of the neck. Look forward.

❷ Inhale your arms to shoulder height, bend the elbows, and bring them to the middle of the chest, palms facing the forehead. Cross the left elbow into the crook of the right elbow. Take the left palm around to press against the right palm, fingers stretching up, thumbs by the nose.

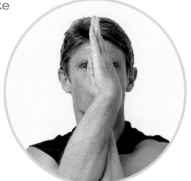

❸ Hold for 30 seconds, palms pressing up and together with each inhalation. Keep the chest broad from sternum to outer rib cage. Repeat on the other side.

89 At the photocopier

❶ Stand tall in Tadasana (page 30) 3ft away from the photocopier (or desk/back of a chair).

❷ Inhaling, take your arms overhead. Release your shoulders down and press the forearms toward each other. Exhaling, pivot from the hips to stretch forward, resting your fingertips on the support.

❸ Shuffle your feet back until knees are over heels, hips over knees. Work for 30 seconds, extending fingertips away from sitting bones equally on both sides, head in line with the spine, looking down to the floor.
Inhale to standing.

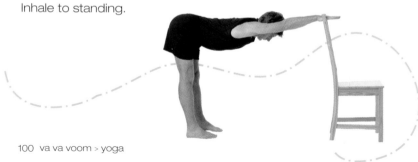

90 Waiting in line

❶ Stand in Tadasana (page 30). Lift your toes and press each one into the floor. Distribute weight evenly between both feet, anchoring equally in the heels and balls.

❷ Bend your right knee, shifting weight onto your left foot. Pull up through the left arch and ankle, back of the knee, and thigh. With hips equal, pelvis tucking up slightly, extend through both sides of the body, shoulders square over hips.

❸ Take your right knee out without moving the hips. Press the right sole into the opposite inner ankle or calf. Hold for 30 seconds, sensing energizing resistance from the straight leg. Repeat on the other leg.

91 Instant 10-second energizer

❶ Tense every muscle in your face and neck: pull up your shoulders, squeeze your eyes, tighten your mouth, screw up your nose, and crease your forehead. Pull in around your ears and back of the scalp, holding the in-breath.

❷ Make your mouth into a wide "O" then an elongated "U," widen your eyes, stretch your ears and throat, and open your cheekbones and jaw to their utmost.

❸ Exhaling, release, feeling your forehead smooth, tongue loose, lips soft and full, and ears relaxed. Look in the mirror and witness how fresh you look.

92 For get-up-and-go

❶ Stand tall in Tadasana (page 30). Bring mind and body into the room, focusing on one point at eye-height.

❷ Bend both knees, hips square and aligned, and shift your weight onto the right leg. Exhaling, lift your left leg over the right thigh. Bend your left knee and wind your shin behind your right calf. Hook your left instep and toes around the right shin to anchor the limb. Check the hips remain level, chest open, shoulders square.

❸ Follow the steps on page 99 to twist your arms into position. Hold for 30 seconds, lengthening the spine with the exhalation. Repeat to the other side.

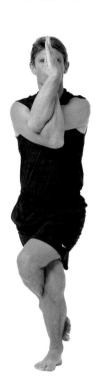

93 Exhilarating shower

To magnify the effects of energizing yoga, purify your body morning and evening with water. In the shower, buff your body with a loofah to cleanse away dead skin cells and bring a sense of invigoration, then direct jets of warm, followed by increasingly bracing cool water to areas you wish to re-energize: patches of cellulite on thighs, buttocks, and upper arms perhaps.

94 Invigorating bath

Mix together 1tsp finely ground black pepper, 1tsp finely grated fresh ginger root, and 3tbsp sea salt. Moisten with water. Take handfuls of this spicy scrub and massage into damp skin, using large strokes in the direction of the heart. Rinse off in the shower, then relax in a hot bath. According to Ayurveda, ginger awakens, kick-starts creativity, and purifies the spirit; black pepper invigorates and detoxifies by boosting circulation and burning ama, toxins.

95 In the heat

❶ Sit comfortably upright, hands resting on knees or thighs. Extend your spine out of the pelvis, close your eyes, and focus on your breathing for a few breath cycles. Feel yourself cooling down.

❷ Roll your tongue up at both sides to form a tube and poke it out through pursed lips. On the inhalation, breathe in slowly through this tube, sucking the air downward as if through a straw.

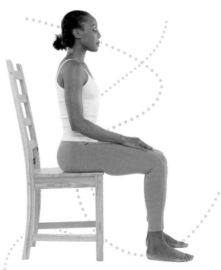

❸ Close the mouth and retain the breath for a few seconds before exhaling through the nostrils. This is 1 cycle. Repeat 5 cycles.

96 Summer energy

❶ In Tadasana (page 30), inhale and step your feet
3–4ft wide, heels and toes parallel, facing forward. Pull
up from ankles to hips, tip the pelvis up slightly,
abdomen back, shoulders over hips, and
extend the spine. Extend the arms out,
palms down.

❷ Turn your left foot out 90°, right
foot in 60°. Exhaling, turn torso and
hips square left. Once stable, inhale, stretch your right arm
up and pivot forward from the hips, placing your right hand
on the left calf, ankle, or floor.

❸ Straighten your left arm up to open your trunk; look at the
thumb. Hold for 30 seconds, revolving the entire trunk with
each inhalation and exhaling into your stable base. Inhale to
standing. Repeat to the right.

97 Generating heat

❶ Sit comfortably upright, hands resting on knees or thighs. Close your eyes and focus on your breathing, feeling it calm and lengthen.

❷ Adopt Vishnu mudra (page 69) with your right hand; raise your hand to your face. Block the left nostril with the ring and little fingers.

❸ Inhale through your right nostril to the count of 4, imagining a warm orange color filling your body. Block the right nostril with the right thumb, retaining the breath for 4. Lift your index and little fingers and exhale through your left nostril to the count of 8. This is 1 cycle. Repeat 5 cycles.

98 Winter warmer

❶ Sit in Vajrasana (page 37). Raise your hips and come on to hands and knees, palms beneath shoulders, fingers facing forward, hips over knees.

❷ Bend forward and place the crown of your head on the floor in front of your fingertips. Tuck your chin toward the throat. Turn the toes under.

❸ Inhaling, take your left shin high on your left tricep; do the same on the right side. Point the feet away from the body, eventually bringing big toes to meet. Hold for 30 seconds or longer, keeping the elbows at 90° to the floor, shins pressing into the arms.

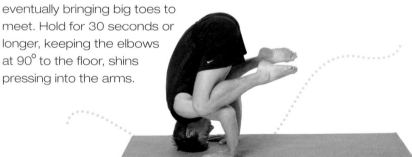

99 Stoking sexual fire

❶ Sit facing your partner. Gaze into each other's eyes, establishing a connection without speech. Savor your lover's look; fill yourself with the sense of his or her presence and energy. Feel that your breathing is quiet and slow, deep in the abdomen.

❷ Let a deep in-breath come naturally, then exhale slowly. Your lover inhales this breath, absorbing your life-force with it.

❸ As your lover exhales, inhale his or her breath, taking within you all his or her essential energy. Continue inhaling and exhaling in this way, setting up a continuous circular breath and energy connection between you.

100 Tapping youthful energy

Perhaps the most energy-draining way to spend a day is with preschoolers. Set up a short impromptu yoga session to focus your energies, divert tantrums, and lift everyone's mood—even the youngest toddlers love it. Here are some starter ideas: sitting in a circle with feet together, flap your knees up and down like a butterfly (see photograph); curl up as tiny seeds then grow into Tree Pose (page 13); lie on your front and come up into Cobra Pose (page 43), hissing at each other; miaou in Cat Pose (page 16) and bark in Dog Pose (page 39); finally, curl up in a ball in Balasana (page 59), taking it in turns to feel the breath coming in and out by placing hands on the back.

101 Finding yourself

In the end it's your unique blend of energies that creates who you are—your personality and temperament, your likes and dislikes, the way you interact with others. Practicing yoga regularly brings your energies into balance to create the best possible expression of who you are. This doesn't just give you a sensational feeling of wellbeing, it allows you to spread good vibes wherever you go.

Acknowledgments

Thanks to all my yoga teachers, especially Nita and Rima Patel.

Resources

Yoga classes
The best way to learn yoga is in a class. Try out a few to help you decide which type of yoga suits you best. For beginners it's often useful to choose a class near your home or workplace: this makes commitment easier.

Books
Yoga: the path to holisitic health, BKS Iyengar,
    Dorling Kindersley 2001
Total Yoga, Nita Patel, MQ Publications 2003
Hot Yoga, Marilyn Barnett, Barron's Educational 2004
The New Book of Yoga, The Sivananda Yoga Centre,
    Ebury 2001